The \
Cure, Dietary
supplement for

Rickets, Osteomalacia,
Osteoporosis, arthritis,
eczema, kidney failure,
Healthy Muscle Function, and
Immune Support.

By

James Dowd

Dedication

This book is dedicated to all those who are afflicted with skin conditions and other chronic illnesses, may they all find relief.

What is vitamin D?

Along with having a number of other biological effects, the group of fat-soluble secosteroids known as vitamin D is in charge of improving the intestinal absorption of calcium, magnesium, and phosphate. The two most crucial compounds in this category for humans are vitamin D3 and vitamin D2.

Vitamin D has to be among the vitamins that science doesn't fully understand.

To begin with, it is a prohormone rather than a vitamin, which means that our body converts it into a hormone. Additionally, there are five separate compounds that make up this substance, with two of them being the most significant to humans. Which are:

D2 vitamin (ergocalciferol).

D3 vitamin (cholecalciferol).

Additionally, research has demonstrated the importance of vitamin D for a variety of vital processes, including calcium absorption, bone formation, and remodeling, immune system modulation, and cell development control.

Vitamin D interacts with our bones, intestines, kidneys, and parathyroid glands to maintain calcium homeostasis throughout the body. Vitamin D receptors are found in our skeletal muscles, skin, lungs, pancreas, and cardiovascular system. In summary, vitamin D is a crucial prohormone for preserving health.

Only 10% of the vitamin D that our bodies require comes from food. When our skin is exposed to sunshine, our bodies create the remaining substances.

What distinguishes vitamin D2 from vitamin D3?

Two significant vitamin D types are vitamin D2 and vitamin D3. D3 is primarily derived from animal sources, while D2 is derived from plants, or it is produced by our bodies when our skin is exposed to sunshine. D3 is more powerful and better absorbed than D2. Because fortified milk and juice are less expensive to produce, they are more likely to include D2.

D2 vitamin

Vitamin D2, commonly referred to as ergocalciferol, is a naturally occurring substance in sun-exposed mushrooms. When exposed to UV light, ergosterol, a yeast component present in mushrooms, changes into ergocalciferol. Maitake mushrooms, which have 786 IU of vitamin D2 per cup, are among the best sources, followed closely by portobello mushrooms (634 IU/cup). Chanterelle mushrooms only contain 114 IU of D2 per cup. A notable source of vitamin D2 that is suitable for vegetarians and vegans is mushrooms.

A synthetic form of vitamin D2 can also be created by irradiating plant and fungal materials that naturally contains ergosterol. Another name for more vitamin D2 is drisdol. Supplementary D2 is less expensive to make than supplemental D3, but it is less stable and less effective at increasing blood levels of vitamin D than synthetic vitamin D3. For vitamin D2 to become active as D3, the body still has to convert it.

D3 vitamin.

Vitamin D3 is produced when the cholesterol in our skin is exposed to sunlight. Trace amounts of vitamin D3 are also present in some animal-derived foods.

7-dehydrocholesterol, a specific type of cholesterol found in our skin, is converted into previtamin D3 when exposed to UVB radiation (wavelength 270-300nm). This is then changed to cholecalciferol in a subsequent process before being activated in the liver and kidneys to produce active vitamin D. Calcitriol, also known as 1,25-dihydroxyvitamin D3, is also known as 1,25(OH)D. (active vitamin D).

Although complicated, the conversion of 7-dehydrocholesterol into active vitamin D3 is rather efficient, and it has been calculated that all it takes to meet our daily requirement of 10 micrograms of vitamin D3 is 10 minutes of summertime exposure to our hands and faces.

Foods including beef liver, cheese, cod liver oil, egg yolks, and fatty fish are naturally high in vitamin D3 (such as mackerel, tuna, and salmon).

Vitamin D3 supplements can be made by taking the cholesterol out of lanolin made from sheep wool and subjecting it to a series of chemical reactions to form 7-dehydrocholesterol. After that, it is exposed to radiation to produce D3 (cholecalciferol). Vegans and vegetarians cannot take supplements manufactured from lanolin, but they can take a D3 supplement created from lichen.

Vitamin D3 is more powerful than D2 and more successfully attaches to vitamin D receptors. Additionally, it is more readily absorbed and transformed into active D.

Before being active in our bodies, all forms of vitamin D2 and D3 received from our diet or through supplements must first undergo conversion in our liver and kidneys.

Vitamin d metabolism flowchart

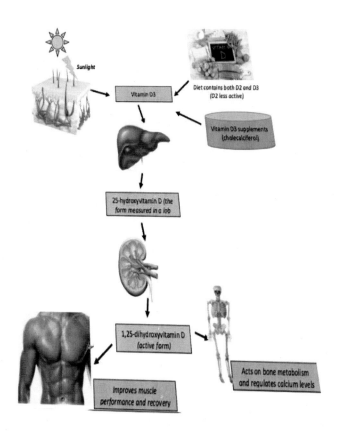

How can I tell if I don't get enough vitamin D?

An assessment of 25(OH)D levels in the blood can be used to identify vitamin D deficiency. Although vitamin D3 has been transformed by the liver to this state, it is still inactive and must undergo additional conversion by the kidneys to produce active vitamin D3, 1,25(OH)D.

It is measured because 25(OH)D is the most stable form of D3. It also persists in the body for several weeks and is the most common form. It is a reliable indicator of how much vitamin D was consumed through diet and sun exposure.

In contrast, 25(OH)D levels are 1,000 times lower and only last for a short time in the body (1,25(OH)D). In times of deficiency and insufficiency, our bodies have a method of increasing the production of active D3 by the kidneys, thus a blood test for 1,25(OH)D may appear normal or high even though your actual levels of vitamin D are low. The 1,25(OH)D test, however, may be employed in some cases with calcium metabolism problems.

Your doctor can determine from your 25(OH)D levels if you have vitamin D deficiency, borderline, sufficient, or toxic levels.

View the flowchart above for a description of the many vitamin d types.

Where can I find vitamin D?

When our skin is exposed to the sun, vitamin D is produced. Supplements containing D2/D3 and foods high in vitamin D can also provide it.

Among the sources of vitamin D2 are:

Mushrooms

Supplements with vitamin D2 (made from irradiated mushrooms and plant material)

Meals with D2 added to them (eg, breakfast cereal, infant formula, margarine, orange juice, milk)

Among the sources of vitamin D3 are:

1. Letting sunlight touch our flesh

2. Butter.

3. Cheese.

4. An egg yolk.

5. Liver.

6. Fish oil and oily fish, such as mackerel, salmon, and tuna.

Supplements for vitamin D3 manufactured from lanolin from sheep's wool.

Lichen-based vitamin D3 pills that are suitable for vegans and vegetarians.

Enhanced D3-containing meals (eg, breakfast cereal, infant formula, margarines, orange juice, and milk).

D2 is the most prevalent type in fortified foods since it is more affordable to produce.

What does having low vitamin D mean?

There is some debate among various professional organizations about what constitutes a low vitamin D level. A vitamin D level gauges blood levels of 25(OH)D. (see the flowchart above for an overview of the different forms vitamin d).

Most professionals advise:

25(OH) D concentrations between 20 and 50 ng/ml: sufficient (good).

12–19 ng/ml range: borderline.

Less than 12 ng/ml levels: Deficiency (low).

Nevertheless, not everyone concurs, and some organizations propose various cut-off values.

According to the Institute of Medicine (IOM)

Amounts greater than 20 ng/ml: Sufficient.

Low levels (20 ng/ml): Deficiency.

Be aware that several IOM committee members publicly stated that excessive testing for vitamin D deficiency was a problem that frequently led to overtreatment. They advocated a lower level of 12.5 ng/ml because they disagreed with a cut-off level of 20 ng/ml for deficiency.

According to the Endocrine Society:

Levels above 30 ng/ml: Sufficient; however, since some assays can be unreliable, levels between 40 and 60 ng/ml would be better able to ensure sufficiency.

21 to 29 ng/ml range: insufficient.

Low levels (20 ng/ml): Deficiency.

Discuss what your doctor deems to be a low vitamin D level with him or her.

What is a lack of vitamin D?

When the levels of vitamin D in your body are below what is considered to be necessary to ensure that all of the processes in your body that depend on vitamin D can work properly, you have a vitamin D insufficiency.

There is disagreement over the threshold for vitamin D deficiency at the moment, with recommendations ranging from less than 20 ng/ml to fewer than 12 ng/ml of 25(OH)D

Is vitamin D soluble in water?

Vitamin D is not fat-soluble. It is thus stored in our adipose (fat) tissue and can occasionally be temporarily mobilized in modest amounts if our daily intake falters. Aside from these, fat-soluble vitamins include vitamins A, E, and K. Since vitamin D is a fat-soluble vitamin, it can become hazardous if ingested in excess.

Vitamin D shortage is common in obese people because more vitamin D is stored in adipose tissue (fat stores) than in the blood, where it may be utilised. Additionally, vitamin D-rich foods and sun exposure are less likely to be consumed by or applied to the skin by obese people.

How does our body make vitamin D?

Although the process of making active vitamin D is quite complicated, it involves sunlight, a particular kind of skin-bound cholesterol, and modification first by the liver and then the kidneys.

A type of cholesterol called 7-dehydrocholesterol is present in our skin. Previtamin D3 is produced when UVB rays with a wavelength in the range of 290 to 315 nm come into contact with 7-dehydrocholesterol. This is then transformed into cholecalciferol and transported to our liver where it is hydroxylated to form calcidiol [25(OH)D]. The kidneys carry out additional hydroxylation to produce 1,25(OH)D (calcitriol), the active form of vitamin D3.

It has been reported that 10 minutes of summer sun exposure on the hands and face is all that is needed to produce the 10 micrograms of vitamin D3 that is considered to be the daily requirement. The entire process of converting 7-dehydrocholesterol into active D3 is quite efficient.

How quickly does the sun produce vitamin D?

The majority of people can easily and reliably get the necessary daily supply of vitamin D thanks to our skin's efficient ability to manufacture the vitamin.

However, for the majority of people, 10 minutes of summertime sun exposure without sunscreen is believed to be adequate. Of course, the amount of time you should spend in the sun depends on your age, skin type, skin tone, the season, and the time of day.

Why does vitamin D levels fall?

Any condition that prevents the body from producing vitamin D from the skin, such as liver or kidney illness, might result in a deficit. Low levels of foods containing vitamin D in the diet or malabsorption diseases can both diminish vitamin D levels.

The ability of our bodies to produce vitamin D may be hampered by the following elements:

1. A chronic condition that makes regular sun exposure impossible.

2. While it is debatable, studies have shown that only Caucasians show a correlation between low vitamin D levels and latitude, living at latitudes above or below 37 degrees north or south of the equator during the winter.

3. Skin tone: People with darker skin produce less vitamin D when exposed to the same amount of sunlight than people with lighter skin.

4. Age: Older people produce less D3 and are less likely to spend time outside in the sun.

5. People (especially women) whose religious practices forbid them from exposing most of their skin and/or faces typically do not get enough sunlight for their skin to produce vitamin D.

6. Sun avoidance and sunscreen use: People spend less time in the sun than in the past due to concerns about skin cancer and skin aging, even though only 10 minutes of summertime direct sunlight is required to produce an adequate daily dose of vitamin D.

Additionally, inadequate dietary intake of vitamin D may also be an influence, but studies have shown that this is not a significant one because less than 10% of the vitamin D in our bodies comes from dietary sources.

The following are other elements that raise the risk of vitamin D deficiency:

1. Long-term liver disease

2. Kidney disease that is ongoing.

3. Emotional eating (eg, anorexia nervosa).

4. Health issues that interfere with the body's ability to absorb vitamin D from food (such as Celiac disease or pancreatic insufficiency).

5. Long-term exclusive breastfeeding or having a mother who is vitamin D deficient when she gives birth.

Obesity

6. (Stores of vitamin D get locked up in adipose tissue).

Using drugs that cause the synthesis or breakdown of vitamin D (such as carbamazepine, efavirenz, phenobarbital, phenytoin, primidone, and rifampin).

LIVER DISEASE

The liver is a small organ, around the size of a football. It is directly below your ribs on the right side of your abdomen. In order to properly digest food and rid your body of hazardous toxins, your liver is essential.

Liver disease may run in families (genetic). Viruses, alcohol use, and obesity are just a few examples of the many factors that can harm the liver and result in liver problems. Cirrhosis, which can cause liver failure and be fatal, is a condition that develops over time as a result of liver damage conditions. But early intervention might give the liver some breathing room.

Liver.

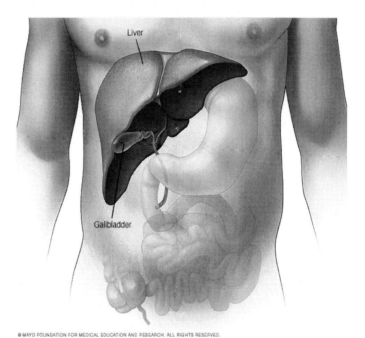

Your largest internal organ is the liver. It is primarily found in the top right corner of your abdomen, above your stomach and around the size of a football.

Symptoms.

There aren't always obvious symptoms and signs of liver disease. If liver disease symptoms do appear, they may include:

1. Yellowish skin tone and eyes (jaundice)

3. Leg and ankle swelling 2. Pain and swelling in the abdomen

4. Skin rashes

5. Urine's deep color

6. Light-colored stool

7. Constant fatigue

8. Vomiting or nauseous

9. Appetite loss

10. Propensity for bruising easily

When to consult a physician.

Make an appointment with your doctor if any symptoms or signs that persist worry you. You should get emergency medical help if your abdominal pain is too severe to allow you to remain still.

Causes.

There are many causes of liver disease.

Infection.

The liver can become infected by parasites and viruses, which results in inflammation and decreased liver function. The viruses that damage the liver can be transmitted through blood or semen, tainted food or water, or direct contact with an infected person. Hepatitis viruses, such as the following, are the most prevalent causes of liver infection:

1 hepatitis A

2. Hepatitis B

3. Hepatitis C

Abnormality in the immune system.

Your liver may be impacted by autoimmune diseases, which occur when your immune system attacks particular body parts. Various autoimmune liver conditions include:

1. Autoimmune liver disease

2. Primary biliary cholangitis

3. Sclerosing cholangiocarcinoma

Genetics.

The buildup of various substances in your liver can result in liver damage if you have an abnormal gene that you either inherited from one of your parents or both of them.

Genetic liver conditions comprise:

1. Hemochromatosis

2. Wilson's illness

3. A lack of alpha-1 antitrypsin

Growths such as cancer

Several examples are:

1. Liver cancer

2. Cancer of the bile ducts

3. A liver tumor

Additional typical causes of liver disease are:

1. Continual alcoholism

2. The liver's accumulation of fat (nonalcoholic fatty liver disease)

3. Specific over-the-counter or prescription drugs

4. Specific herbal substances

Risk elements

You may be more vulnerable to developing liver disease if you have:

1. Abuse of alcohol

2. Obesity

3. Type 2 diabetes

4. Body art or piercings

5. Utilizing shared needles when injecting drugs

6. before 1992, blood transfusions

7. Being exposed to the blood and bodily fluids of others

8. Unguarded sex

9. Being exposed to specific toxins or chemicals

10. Liver disease in the family

Complications.

Depending on the root of your liver issues, there are different liver disease complications. Untreated liver disease may develop into liver failure, a condition that poses a serious risk to life.

Prevention

To stop liver illness:

1. Use alcohol sparingly. That entails up to one drink per day for women and up to two drinks per day

for men for healthy adults. More than eight drinks per week for women and more than 15 drinks per week for men is considered heavy or high-risk drinking.

2. Refrain from taking risks. When having sex, use a condom. If you decide to get a tattoo or have your body pierced, be picky about the shop's cleanliness and safety. If you use illegal intravenous drugs, get help. If you inject drugs, don't share needles.

Obtain a vaccine. Consult your doctor about receiving the hepatitis A and hepatitis B vaccines if you have a higher risk of developing hepatitis or if you have already had the virus in any form.

3. Use drugs responsibly. Only take prescription and over-the-counter medications as directed and only when necessary. Don't combine booze with prescription drugs. Before combining herbal supplements with prescription or

over-the-counter medications, consult your doctor.

4. Steer clear of bodily fluids and blood from other individuals. Accidental needle jabs and poor handling of blood or bodily fluids can transmit hepatitis viruses.

5. Maintain food safety. Before consuming food or preparing it, fully wash your hands. Use bottled water when visiting a developing nation, wash your hands frequently, and brush your teeth.

6. Use aerosol sprays with caution. Wear a mask and use these products in an area that is well-ventilated when applying paint, insecticides, fungicides, or other hazardous substances. Always adhere to the manufacturer's guidelines.

7. Keep your skin safe. Wear gloves, long sleeves, a hat, and a mask when using insecticides and other hazardous chemicals to prevent

chemical absorption through your skin.

8. Keep a suitable weight. Non-alcoholic fatty liver disease can result from obesity.

Diagnosis.

Treatment should be based on the cause and severity of liver impairment. Your doctor will probably begin by taking a thorough medical history and physical examination.

Your physician might then suggest:

Blood analysis. A group of blood tests known as liver function tests can be used to diagnose liver disease. Additional blood tests can be run to look for particular liver problems or hereditary diseases.

Scanning tests MRI, CT, and ultrasound scans can reveal liver damage.

A tissue sample is examined. A tissue sample (biopsy) from your liver may be collected in order to diagnose liver disease and look for indicators of liver damage. During a liver biopsy, a large needle is often used to remove tissue samples from the liver that are subsequently submitted to a lab for analysis.

Treatment.

Your diagnosis will determine how to treat your liver condition. Some liver conditions can be managed with lifestyle changes, such as giving up alcohol or losing weight, usually as part of a medical plan that also includes careful liver function monitoring. Other liver issues might need surgery or medication treatment.

A liver transplant may eventually be needed as treatment for liver disease that causes or has caused liver failure.

Home remedies and way of life.

Your liver health can frequently be improved by changing some of your lifestyle habits. If you have been given a liver disease diagnosis, your doctor might advise you to:

1. Use alcohol only occasionally, if at all.

2. Steer clear of foods containing high-fructose corn syrup, Tran's fats, processed carbohydrates, and red meat.

3. Work out at a moderate intensity for 30 to 60 minutes three to four times per week.

4. If you are overweight, reduce your daily calorie intake by 500 to 1,000 calories.

Various forms of medicine.

There is no alternative medicine treatment for liver disease that has been proven effective. Although some studies have suggested potential advantages, more research is required.

However, some nutritional and herbal supplements can be detrimental to your liver. Liver disease has been linked to more than a thousand prescription drugs and natural remedies, including:

1. A vitamin

2. Ma-huang

3. Germander

4. Mistletoe

4. Mistletoe

6. Chaparral

6. Chaparral

8. Comfrey

8. Comfrey

10. Pennyroyal oil, no. 10

Before using any additional or alternative medicines, it's crucial to discuss the potential hazards with your doctor in order to safeguard your liver.

Getting ready for a meeting.

You might be directed to a medical professional who focuses in the liver (hepatologist).

How you can conduct.

1. Recognize any prerequisites, such as the need to skip solid food the day before your appointment.

2. Jot down all of your symptoms, even those that might not seem to be connected to the reason you made the appointment.

3. Create a list of all the vitamins, supplements, and prescriptions you use.

4. List all of your important medical information, including any other conditions.

5. Jot down important personal details, such as any recent changes or sources of stress in your life.

6. Invite a friend or family member to go with you so you can remember what the doctor says.

7. Make a list of inquiries to make to your physician.

Inquiries to make to your physician.

1. What is the most probable reason for my symptoms?

2. What types of tests do I require? Are there any special preparations needed for these exams?

3. Are my liver issues likely to be short-term or chronic?

4. What medical procedures are offered?

5. Should I stop using a particular supplement or medication?

6. Should I give up drinking alcohol?

7. I have additional medical issues. How can I combine management of these conditions?

8. Do my kids have a liver disease risk?

Don't be afraid to ask your doctor additional questions at your appointment in addition to the ones you've prepared.

What signs of vitamin D deficiency are there?

The majority of people do not know they are deficient in vitamin D until their doctor orders a blood test to check for it. The symptoms of vitamin D deficiency are initially vague. Any symptoms that reflect how vitamin D affects your immune system, mood, and bone health include:

1. Back or bone pain

2. Persistent exhaustion or fatigue

3. Continual infections (such as colds or flu)

4. Alopecia

5. Depression or a bad mood

6. Achy muscles

Osteoporosis

Osteoporosis

8. Bad oral hygiene

9. Skin injuries that are slow to heal.

More obvious symptoms, such as bone fractures, rickets, or osteomalacia, may manifest if the deficiency persists untreated.

Low vitamin D levels in the blood have also been linked to

1. Memory and cognitive impairment in older people

Cancer

2. (Particularly colon cancer)

3. Cardiovascular illness and a higher chance of dying from a heart attack or a stroke

4. Kidney illness

5. Children with severe asthma.

Additionally, research indicates that vitamin D may help treat or prevent a number of other disorders, including diabetes, high blood pressure, and multiple sclerosis.

Describe Rickets.

When children have rickets, a bone condition, their bones become softer and weaker. It is caused by a prolonged lack of vitamin D, which prevents the body from absorbing other minerals like calcium and phosphate, which are essential for healthy bones. The term "osteomalacia" refers to the softening of adult bones.

Children between the ages of six and 36 months are the ones that contract rickets most frequently. Although uncommon in the United States, it is widespread elsewhere, particularly in parts of Asia where vegetarianism and short daylight hours are common.

Being born to a mother who is vitamin D-deficient, exclusively breastfeeding, having poor nutrition, not getting enough sun exposure, and having malabsorption syndromes that prevent nutrient absorption are risk factors. Dark-skinned children who reside in cloudy northern cities or those whose cultural or religious beliefs forbid exposure to the sun are also at an increased risk of developing the condition.

Infantile rickets symptoms include:

1. A delay in the skull's bones closing up

2. Bowed legs and knock-knees from the ends of the long bones being larger.

3. Bead-like nodules where the rib cage's bones attach to cartilage.

4. Chest deformity brought on by the ribs' pressure on the diaphragm

5. Failure to sit up or walk on time

6. Poor growth

7. Sleep issues

8. Agitation

9. A thinned or swollen skull;

10. Tooth decay and inadequate tooth growth

Bone fractures, convulsions, muscle spasms, and mental retardation can also happen in really severe cases.

Rickets can also strike nursing women who consume inadequate amounts of vitamin D in their diets. Aches and pains in the muscles, bones, and joints, as well as fatigue and hair loss, may be symptoms.

Supplementing with vitamin D is a common part of treatment, even after symptoms have subsided. Calcium intravenously may also be administered in severe cases. In some cases, surgery may be necessary to fix distorted bones and muscles.

What is vitamin D's purpose?

The majority of people are aware of the benefits of vitamin D for healthy bones and calcium absorption, but vitamin D is also necessary for numerous other essential bodily functions.

Vitamin D deficiency has been linked to:

1. Memory and cognitive decline in older people

2. Muscle, back, or bone discomfort

Cancer

3. (Particularly colon cancer)

4. Cardiovascular disease and a higher chance of dying from a heart attack or a stroke

5. Constant exhaustion and fatigue

6. Continual infections (such as colds and flu)

7. Alopecia

8. Kidney illness

9. Depression or a bad mood

10. Osteomalacia

11. Osteoporosis

12. Poor dental health

13. Rickets

14. Children with severe asthma

15. Skin injuries that take a long time to heal.

Who needs to have their vitamin D levels checked?

The majority of professionals oppose widespread vitamin D insufficiency testing. This is due to:

1. Tests for vitamin D are significantly more expensive than supplementation.

2. Routine screening can result in overtreatment of perceived vitamin D insufficiency

3. There is no agreed-upon unambiguous cut-off point for deficiency.

Even if they don't exhibit any symptoms, most doctors advise giving vitamin D supplements to babies, kids, and adults who are at high risk of vitamin D insufficiency without first doing a deficiency test.

When someone is suspected of having significant vitamin D insufficiency, testing may be necessary. In these situations, it is also important to look into the renal function, calcium, phosphate, and alkaline phosphatase blood levels, as well as other tests.

Testing for vitamin D is recommended for those who have:

1. Low serum levels of calcium or phosphate or an inexplicable rise in alkaline phosphatase

2. Uncommon osteoporosis

3. Older people who experience unexplained limb discomfort near a joint

4. Unusual fractures, unexplained discomfort in the bones, or other signs of metabolic bone disease.

If it is determined that a person has a metabolic bone disease rather than a straightforward vitamin D deficiency, they may need to be sent to a specialist.

What dosage of vitamin D should I use?

There is some disagreement about whether people should take vitamin D supplements or increase their level of sun exposure while still using sun safety precautions.

Only a small amount of vitamin D is found in our diet because most of it is produced by sunshine, which makes up around 90% of the vitamin D in our bodies. Infants, young children, people with physical or mental disabilities, people with malabsorption disorders, the elderly, and those who cover their skin for religious or cultural reasons are more susceptible to vitamin D insufficiency than other groups of people.

The required amount of vitamin D per day is:

1. 400 IU from birth to one year old

2. 600 IU for people aged 1 to 70.

3. Over 70 years of age: 800 IU

For individuals, 4,000 IU/day of vitamin D is the healthy top level. However, despite the fact that higher doses are not advised, doctors may nonetheless offer them for patients who are vitamin D deficient. For children, the top limit is 1000IU for newborns up to 6 months, 2,500IU for toddlers up to 3 years, 3,000IU for kids between 4 and 8 years old, and 4,000IU for kids over 9 years old. When using high amounts of vitamin D, blood levels should be checked.

The Endocrine Society, a reputable institution, advises somewhat greater safe maximum limits and daily vitamin D consumption. This group focuses on helping those who are more susceptible to deficiencies, including as transplant recipients, persons with long-term health issues that can lead to malabsorption, and people using medications that could endanger their bone health.

Currently, recommendations do not distinguish between using different types of vitamin D supplements (such as D2 or D3).

What amount of vitamin D is excessive?

Although it is uncommon, vitamin D toxicity can occur if you take too many supplements. Neither exposure to the sun nor consumption of foods containing vitamin D can cause vitamin D poisoning.

When blood levels of 25(OH)D rise above 150 ng/ml (375 nmol/L), vitamin D toxicity is thought to develop. Even if you stop taking supplements, levels of vitamin D may take several weeks to return to normal because it is a fat-soluble vitamin.

Early signs of vitamin D toxicity include nausea, vomiting, constipation/diarrhea, weakness, or frequent urination and are brought on by having too much calcium in the blood (hypercalcemia), which is linked to vitamin D levels and calcium absorption. Long-term exposure to levels that are too high can result in kidney stones made of calcium, bone discomfort, headaches, sleepiness, and itching. Extremely high amounts may also result in low blood levels of vitamin K2, which paradoxically may result in calcium loss from the bones. There are claims that high vitamin D levels have led to renal failure.

Treatment for vitamin D toxicity involves ceasing vitamin D tablets and limiting calcium intake. Additionally, fluids and other drugs like bisphosphonates may be administered.

According to studies, using 40,000–60,000 IU of vitamin D daily for a few months can be harmful. However, this is a lot more than the 4,000 IU/day for adults that is considered the safe upper limit for vitamin D. For most adults, the Recommended Dietary Allowance (RDA) for vitamin D is 600 IU per day.

Before using vitamin and mineral supplements, always see your doctor.

How vegan is vitamin D?

In the past, sheep wool lanolin was used to make vitamin D3, but recently a vegan/vegetarian form of the vitamin has become available. This version, known as Vitashine, is made from lichen, a type of plant typically found on rocks, walls, or trees. Additionally, this product is free of dairy, wheat, gluten, and sugar.

Supplements for vitamin D2 made by irradiating mushrooms are also suitable for vegans and vegetarians.

Studies have revealed that D3 significantly raises blood levels of vitamin D compared to D2.

What dishes contain vitamin D?

Foods containing vitamin D are rare. Both foods and dietary supplements contain either D2 or D3 forms of vitamin D.

The following foods contain vitamin D2:

1. Mushrooms

2. Foods that have been D2 fortified (e.g., breakfast cereal, infant formula, margarine, orange juice, milk)

Vitamin D3 can be obtained from:

1. Butter

2. Cheddar

3. Egg white

4. Liver

5. Fish oil and oily fish (such as mackerel, salmon, and tuna)

6. D3-enriched fortified foods (eg, breakfast cereal, infant formula, margarines, orange juice, milk)

D2 is the most prevalent type in fortified foods since it is more affordable to produce.

Why is milk given a vitamin D boost?

In the United States, milk began receiving vitamin D in the late 1930s. Before that time, rickets was a prevalent illness that disproportionately affected impoverished children residing in dirty and industrialized American cities.

Rickets is a bone disease that mainly affects young children and results in growth and bone abnormalities. It was initially identified as a disease in 1650. Cod liver oil wasn't initially given for rickets until 1824, despite the fact that it had long been used as a remedy for other illnesses. Researchers were able to isolate active vitamin D in the 1930s thanks to a seminal 1922 study that demonstrated how adding whole milk or cod liver oil to the diets of malnourished children with rickets may cure them.

Initially, adding vitamin D to milk required either irradiating it or giving it to cows together with irradiated yeast. The more straightforward and efficient technique of blending vitamin D concentrate with milk was introduced in the 1940s, nevertheless, and it is being used today.

Thanks for Reading

Manufactured by Amazon.ca
Acheson, AB

15700846R00035